Changing bad habit to a good habit

By

William T. Carlson

Table of content

Copyright

Introduction

Chapter 1

What is bad habit?

What Is the Average Time to Break a Bad Habit?

Why Is Breaking a Bad Habit So Difficult?

How to Quit Bad Behaviors.

Chapter 2

The Effect of Habit

Chapter 3

How many emotions manifest themselves in your brain and how simple it is to modify them?

How to handle unpleasant feelings.

Chapter4

ways to assist someone in overcoming a bad habit.

Chapter 5

Creating habits that help you achieve your goal.

Conclusion

Exercise cultivates habits.

Introduction

A routine of conduct that is performed on a regular basis that frequently happens unconsciously is referred to as a habit (or wont in a funny and formal sense).

A habit was described as "a more or less established manner of thinking, willing, or feeling formed via previous repetition of a mental experience" in The American Journal of Psychology (1903). Habitual behavior frequently goes unnoticed by those who engage in it since it is unnecessary to conduct self-analysis when performing everyday chores. Habits can sometimes be required. In a study of daily experience conducted in 2002, habit researcher Wendy Wood and her colleagues discovered that over 43% of daily behaviors are carried out out of habit. Through the process of habit formation, new behaviors might become automatic. The behavioral patterns that people repeat become imprinted in neural circuits, making it difficult to break old habits and difficult to build new ones, although it is possible to create new habits through repetition.

There is a gradual improvement in the relationship between the context and the action when behaviors are repeated in a reliable setting. As a result, the behavior becomes more automatic in such a situation. All or more of the following characteristics of automatic behavior include efficiency, lack of awareness, unintentionality, and uncontrollability.

Everybody has bad habits. No matter if you frequently talk with your mouth full, bite your nails, or procrastinate endlessly, negative habits are detrimental to our ideas of who we want to be and how we see ourselves.

The issue is that, because of how our brains are built, routines and habits are formed out of our daily encounters. Our brain can focus on other things when specific tasks, like riding a bike, operating a vehicle, or tying our shoes, are done automatically. The development of routines and habits isn't necessarily a bad thing. A poor habit can, however, be formed just as easily as a good one. Additionally, they can be quite hard to break.

I'm going to get into the psychology of how to overcome unhealthy behaviors

in this essay. I'm going to examine what causes harmful habits from the very beginning before outlining a simple three-step process for getting rid of negative habits and replacing them with better ones.

Chapter 1

What is a bad habit?

A bad habit is an unfavorable pattern of behavior. Examples of common ones are procrastination, excessive spending, and nail-biting. A poor habit is a consistent behavior pattern that you believe is negatively affecting a particular aspect of your life. A negative habit is one that is repeated frequently and differs from an addiction or mental disease in terms of how it affects willpower.

In general, if you are able to "break" a negative behavior with willpower, it was just that—a habit. If you are unable to utilize willpower to change a harmful habit, you probably have some

type of addiction or a mental disorder of some kind.While many behaviors are commonly accepted to be harmful habits, such as smoking, binge drinking, and teeth grinding, what you may view as a negative habit may be totally logical to someone else, and vice versa. For instance, you might think that "viewing too much television" is a negative habit that you'd like to kick, but for someone who is just beginning a course on writing for television, watching a lot of it is par for the course. Similar to how you might want to "spend less time on your phone," a person who runs their business on their phone may not want to do so. This is the complete opposite of what they want to be doing, whether

it's maintaining their brand's social media profiles or sending emails and texts nonstop.

What Is the Average Time to Break a Bad Habit?

Since it was initially established, the widely held notion that it takes 21 days to form or break a habit has come under ongoing criticism. Give each new component you introduce to your morning routine a fair chance, as we mentioned in my book on morning routines. It is insufficient to give anything a try for a short period of time before giving up. Despite the fact that opinions on how long something takes to become a habit vary, we advise giving each new component at least a

one-to two-week trial to see if you like it. With that stated, I think the 21-day guideline is a reasonable one to use, as long as you don't lose hope if you can't overcome a certain habit in this precise amount of time. Think of the 21-day rule as a guideline rather than a precise calculation.

Why Is Breaking a Bad Habit So Difficult?

It can be challenging to try to kick a negative habit when you've been doing it day in and day out, week in and week out, year in and year out. Negative behavior is kind of rooted in who you are. Remember the following 21-day "rule"? The reality is that the habit you are trying to break has probably been

with you for some time; probably many months, years, and possibly even decades. It may take you exactly 21 days, 42 days, or more to break a particular habit.

It seems logical that trying to change a negative habit in a short period of time will be challenging if you have been doing it every day for many years. However, it is not impossible to do so, and that is what the remainder of this essay will discuss. Over the years, I've been able to break a lot of unhealthy habits, like eating less fast food, staring at devices less, and finding an exercise routine that suits my lifestyle.

But I'm still a long way from finishing my quest to develop healthy habits. I'm

always trying to find ways to maximize my energy and live a better life. It's likely that if you're reading this, you, too, have certain habits that you'd like to modify. So why is it so tough to form new habits in general? Due to the

lack of a mechanism to assist you in completing the task (unless you've reached the problematic tipping point of acquiring an addiction or diagnosable disease), Even then, the procedures in place are only intended to assist you in breaking the bad habit; they do not provide you with the means to start new, healthier ones.

What causes this to occur? partially because of the persistent myth that those who battle addiction or mental

health concerns are somehow different from the rest of us "regular" people. This is not only incorrect, but it's also quite dangerous since it makes people who are struggling feel even more ashamed and stigmatized, which discourages them from getting treatment.

How to Quit Bad Behavior

Humans are basic beings. We don't want much more from life than to continue doing the things we enjoy doing and to avoid doing the things we don't. Unfortunately, living in a way where we never feel uncomfortable is not only impractical, but would also swiftly turn into its own form of confinement.

With that positive mindset in mind, keep reading to find out a simple three-step process for breaking negative behaviors and replacing them with better ones:

1. **Identify the behavior you would like to change, together with its stimuli.** Good and unhealthy habits alike are established through repetition. it's essential for us to first identify the

repetition before ceasing it in order to stop a harmful habit. once you wake up, you immediately head to the restroom, wash your teeth, placed on your gym clothes, sit right down to meditate, or start the kettle to brew your favorite cup of tea or coffee. The first step in attempting to break a

negative habit is to identify what it is right before you engage in it.

However, let's take a quick step back. Asking yourself why you would like to break (or change) this behavior in the first place will help you to truly be able to do so. For instance, if you are a chronic procrastinator who hardly ever completes anything because your focus is constantly diverted, you'll tell yourself that if you can kick the habit, you will be more productive in the long run, opening up more opportunities,

making more connections, and (probably) putting extra money in the bank. If you've smoked your entire life, tell yourself ahead of your face that quitting might potentially add years to

your life, years that you simply could actually watch your children, grandchildren, or maybe great-grandchildren grow and mature.

List the subsequent factors that occur right before you engage in the negative behavior in question, after you've got determined why you wish to break it. Do these triggers operate their own, or are they a component of a much bigger behavioral pattern?

It's time to move on to finding a replacement for your poor behavior once you have your reasons for wanting to change this habit, the

stimuli that drive you to try to to this habit, and any bigger perspective of how these factors operate together.

2. **Choose a replacement for Your Bad Habit:** Understanding the way to break a bad habit, however, also entails understanding that you simply frequently can't just "break" a terrible habit; too often, you would like to substitute it with something else.

This has a simple justification. Returning to the concept of stimuli and habit stacks, your brain develops an expectation that your negative habit are going to be carried out when you build one habit on top of another or observe a trigger that signals it is time to engage in it. you'll feel compelled to engage in this terrible habit right now, but it'll be challenging to resist

because there is nothing to replace it

with. However, by replacing your bad habit with an honest one, you'll prevent the habit stack from being broken and give your brain something to do when it encounters the trigger that led to your old behavior.

To better illustrate my point, here is an example: lets say you've started to go out for a drink or two every evening after work. After an extended week, visiting a bar with a few pals on a Friday night was just a casual start to this. Soon you discover that, whether or not you've got guests, you perform this ritual every evening. although this once-in-a-while incident has now become a full-fledged habit, you're still having a good time.

You are concerned about what might

occur if you let this terrible habit persist.

You join up for a gym membership and start going there after work instead, realizing that quitting the negative habit of visiting a pub after work and just going home instead is unlikely to last. In doing so, you maintain the ritual of unwinding during a location that serves as a transition between work and home while also ensuring that your body experiences a favorable outcome.

Your choice of a replacement for a problematic habit will depend on both the habit and your personal preferences. this is often the same concept as the example that smokers need something to do with their hands after quitting smoking, which you'll

have heard or experienced. Once you've replaced the unhealthy habit with a healthy alternative, you will be well on your way to breaking it for good.

3.Plan for failure, aim for fulfillment: Your attitude and level of readiness will determine the ultimate stage in learning how to break a harmful habit.

Even once you feel like the odds are stacked against you, you want to have faith in your ability to overcome a negative habit in order to succeed. you want to be tenacious in your efforts to break the habit, but you want to also be patient with yourself and the

process. you want to view the 21-day "rule" as a recommendation rather than an exact scientific calculation, as I stated earlier during this post. it'll take longer to change a habit, the more embedded it's in your life.

This is what I mean when I say, "Plan for failure, aim for fulfillment ." you want to treat yourself when you reach even the smallest of milestones (one day, two days, three days without engaging within the harmful habit). you would like to picture yourself permanently kicking this harmful behavior. The mechanism for slip-ups (or near slip-ups) which may otherwise make you feel like you're starting over must be in place, though, so as to avoid this feeling.

I advise joining a support group, either online or—if your bad habit may be a common one—in person, where you'll share tips with others who are struggling to break the same bad habit as you while also working to support each other toward letting go of this habit completely. While this would possibly not be necessary for every bad habit you wish to break, for the larger , stickier habits, i like to recommend doing so.

When you set goals for success but prepare for failure, you create sure you're providing yourself every opportunity to handle disappointment. you begin to think differently as a result of an emotional reaction. as an example , researchers have discovered

that folks typically recall sad memories when they are depressed but good ones when they are upbeat. Another illustration would be that when people are frightened, they often begin to scan their surroundings for other threats and are more inclined to entertain thoughts of other terrifying things. On the opposite hand, when an individual is content, they often take notice of more pleasant things throughout the day.

The final stage of an emotional reaction is when you start to feel a desire to act differently than how you typically do. As an example, when you're upset, you would possibly want to yell at someone or engage in combat. Or, if you're terrified, you'll

have a strong need to flee. Or, if you are feeling down, you would possibly just want to stay at home by yourself and isolate yourself in your room.

How are you able to tell what emotion you are experiencing?

We frequently wish to comprehend our emotional responses after experiencing them. have you ever ever struggled to identify your emotions? Sometimes it can be difficult to grasp our feelings because they can be so complex. this is often due, in part, to the very fact that the same emotion can occasionally feel different in other contexts. as an example , fear of a lion might not feel the same as fear of giving a speech in front of your class.

the very fact that many emotional states can occasionally feel similar adds to the complexity of sentiments. as an example , both fear and anger can cause you to tremble and increase your heart rate.

Therefore, you continue to need to identify the emotion you are experiencing when you become aware of it. as an example , you would possibly feel as though a lion is in front of you, your heart is thrashing rapidly, and you desperately want to escape . After considering several emotions you would possibly be experiencing, you would possibly determine that "fear" is your best bet. you would possibly be thinking, "I'm actually feeling fear immediately because I am

afraid the lion could hurt me," or something similar. However, during a terrifying circumstance like this, you would possibly not even be aware of your fear until you run away and give it some time to sink in. Scientists have discovered that some people have a harder time identifying their emotions than others. people that have a hard time comprehending their emotions often have a harder time improving their own feelings.

Chapter 2

The Effect of Habit

Given that habits are your brain's way of conserving energy and that you spend roughly 6 of your 16 waking hours doing things you're not aware of, it might be worthwhile to understand what goes on here.

Duhigg found that each one habits, including drinking coffee every morning, have an easy 3-part loop at their core.

The cue is what prompts you to hold out the habit, like setting the alarm at 7 a.m.

every morning and eating breakfast at the table .

The habit is that the behavior you then

naturally exhibit, which, for sipping coffee, could also be to head over to press the "large cup" button on your coffeemaker and turn it on.

The rich aroma smell of your coffee, its hearty flavor, and therefore the chance to watch the steam rising up from the cup as it sits on your kitchen table in the sunlight are all rewards for completing the routine. are you able to tell I really love coffee?

During this loop, your brain's activity only increases twice. Both at the start and the conclusion, when the association between cue and routine is strengthened (here may be a visual from the book).

Why not reinforce it?

Aha!

This is how habits are formed, and therefore the more strongly this relationship develops, the harder it is to break them. But it's still possible. By changing the routine, the sole component of the loop, you'll alter your behaviors.

Naturally, a habit becomes more ingrained in your brain the more times you reinforce it.

In the instance of coffee, you would possibly have a craving as soon as you sit down at your kitchen table, and if the machine is broken and you cannot make any that day, you'll likely become really irate and buy some later at work.

The key to breaking a habit is to vary the routine while leaving everything else alone. Your most vital habit is willpower, which you'll gradually improve in three different ways.

Willpower, consistent with Duhigg, is far and away one of the most crucial habits because it improves our performance in every area of life. Not all habits are created equal.

I don't want to urge you to eat well, get enough sleep, and exercise frequently because I've done studies on willpower to the moon and back. Colin, a buddy of mine, excels therein area.

Here are three unusual techniques to gradually increase your overall willpower capacity instead:

1. **Do something that demands plenty of self-control.** A difficult wake-up schedule or a stringent diet, as an example , will force you to practice delaying pleasure continually and provides you more willpower to use throughout the rest of the day.

2. **Consider worst-case scenarios beforehand** . you will not lose your cool if you merely imagine your boss yelling at you before it actually happens.

3. **Keep your independence.** I discovered the opposite day that having liberty was crucial to leading a passionate life. I discovered today that if you're taking it away, your willpower also vanishes. Your willpower muscle gets tired much more quickly when you have to do duties that have been given to you by another person.

Chapter 3

How many emotions manifest themselves in your brain and how simple it is to modify them?

Recent imaging research suggests that a series of modifications to the limbic and cognitive control circuitry occur because the emotional brain develops.

Adolescence may be a time when these changes are most noticeable since there may be a greater need for self-control in a range of emotional and social situations.

What occurs when an emotion is genuinely triggered? Scientists have discovered that an "emotional reaction" actually consists of a spread of components.

The brain alters what's happening in the body as part of an emotional reaction. as an example , you would possibly feel your heart begin to race and your breathing quicken when you're scared or angry. Or, if you are feeling melancholy, your eyes can start to shred . Some muscles in your body may contract reflexively thanks to emotions. as an example , once you are happy, you would possibly not even be aware that you are smiling, your speech might sound more animated, and you would possibly stand up a little taller. it is important to pay attention to your feelings and to practice identifying them. you will be able to solve difficulties and recover from illnesses more quickly if you do

this. It also helps to reflect on past instances of sadness, fear, and anger and ask yourself what you've got learned from them and how you would respond if a similar circumstance arose in the future.

Regarding bad feelings

Any emotion that creates you unhappy and wretched is referred to as a negative emotion. These feelings cause you to despise both yourself and people , which lowers your level of self-assurance, self-worth, and overall life pleasure.

Negative emotions like hate, rage, jealousy, and despair are common. However, these emotions are entirely normal within the appropriate situation.

counting on how long we allow negative emotions to affect us and how we choose to express them, they'll reduce our zest for life.

Negative feelings kept inside cause a downward spiral.

We are unable to objectively think, act, or view circumstances from their actual perspective once we are experiencing negative emotions. When this happens, we often see and recall just the things we wanted to see. This simply makes the anger or grief last longer and keeps us from fully appreciating life.

The issue gets more complicated the longer this continues. Inappropriately managing negative emotions can

sometimes be damaging, like when rage is expressed violently.

Complex reactions are emotions.

Emotions are intricate bodily reactions involving numerous biochemical and physiological processes. We enter an aroused state as a results of the hormones and chemicals that our brain releases in response to our thoughts. this is often how all feelings, whether good or bad, are created. It's a complicated process, and frequently we lack the tools to deal with unpleasant emotions. We struggle to deal with them because of this when we encounter them.

How to handle unpleasant feelings

There are several coping mechanisms available to deal with unpleasant feelings. These consist of:

1. **Don't** overthink situations by going over them repeatedly in your mind.

2. Try to be rational, acknowledge that unpleasant emotions can happen from time to time, and consider measures to improve your mood.

3. Use relaxing activities to unwind, such as reading, walking, or conversing with a friend.

4. In order to be ready in advance, learn to recognize how sadness, loss, and rage make you feel and which circumstances cause them.

5. Exercise: Aerobic activity reduces your stress hormone levels and improves your ability to handle unpleasant emotions.

6. Letting go of the past will free you to live in the present and will prevent you from becoming mired in regret.

Chapter4

ways to assist someone in overcoming a bad habit.

Do you know anyone attempting to kick a bad habit? Perhaps your wife wants to stop eating five cookies after dinner, or perhaps your spouse wants to stop biting his nails. Or maybe your closest buddy realizes that her family gets frustrated by her habit of frequently checking her phone and decides it's time to cut back. There are things you may do to encourage a loved one who has decided to try to kick a bad habit.

Condemn judgment.

Maintain objectivity by talking about

habits rather than individuals.Instead of referring to the knuckle cracking as a general characteristic of the person, talk about it specifically.

ID causes

Determine whether certain circumstances tend to set off the undesirable behavior. Keep a notebook or journal with information about the time, place, and feelings connected to the harmful behavior.

Take little steps

Start by establishing manageable, modest goals. For instance, your spouse can set a goal to refrain from biting his nails for the next five minutes when he feels the need to do so. Increase the time gradually after he

is capable of doing that.

Adjust your attention

Encourage them to think of the positive rather than the negative—what they are giving up. In addition to being a healthier habit, going for a stroll after dinner is more enjoyable and something you can do with your family.

erect barriers

Make the bad habit harder to maintain by putting the phone in a pocket that is difficult to access or keeping the cookies on a different floor of your home.

Fill the space.

Encourage your buddy to replace the temptation to check her phone for the

twelfth time in two minutes with a constructive habit, such as taking four long, cleansing breaths.

Be persistent.

Many behaviors are ingrained habits that are difficult to break. Don't lecture or nag your loved one if you notice them slipping. Instead, practice empathy and try to comprehend how challenging it might be to alter a behavior that frequently happens automatically.

Amplify the good.

Note admirable efforts and rejoice in whatever degree of success there may be.

The majority of bad habits are

generally harmless acts that we would prefer not to engage in. Compulsive habits, which people are unable to quit, even when they wish to, are at the other end of the spectrum. Consult a mental health professional for an assessment and potential treatment if you or someone you know is experiencing distress or impairment as a result of an uncontrollable behavior.

Chapter 5

Creating habits that help you achieve your goals.

1.Set clear objectives.

Sadly, lacking a clear finish line is one of the things that prevents many goal-setters from reaching their objectives. The phrase "reduce weight" is ambiguous; is one pound considered a victory?

As an alternative, those who consistently achieve their objectives tend to be quite specific in what they hope to accomplish, such as "reduce 10 pounds in 3 months."

2. **Make time to work on your objectives**.

Time doesn't carve itself out, as successful people are aware of. If they are serious about achieving a goal, they set aside a particular amount of time to focus on it. They treat these sessions with the same respect they would if they were working with clients. When you have the routine of setting aside time to work towards your goals, you'll always achieve them.

3. **Prioritize smaller goals while pursuing the larger one.**

Many people begin with lofty objectives that motivate them but are, regrettably, difficult to achieve. It's crucial to divide large goals into

smaller "milestone" objectives so that you can monitor your progress and maintain motivation as you move toward them.

4. **Acknowledge that every quality can be enhanced.**

Some people become demoralized and give up because they believe they aren't capable of achieving their goals. Those who succeed understand that this is untrue; even IQ or personality can develop with time. You'll succeed more quickly if you make it a habit to improve all of your traits.

5. **Be persistent at all times.**

The adage "When the going gets tough, the tough get going" is a way of life for individuals who routinely succeed in

their aims. They mentally get ready to push through by acknowledging how challenging the road to their objectives will be. If you want to be someone who achieves their goals, having the habit of endurance is crucial.

6. **Outline your goals.**

Successful people have a strong practice of keeping a written record of every goal they set and the date it was attained. In addition to giving them a track record to build on, this makes the objective seem more achievable.

7. Substitute good habits for bad ones.

Setting a goal to do something new is far more beneficial than setting a goal to quit doing something. If you want to break a bad habit, concentrate on

developing a new behavior for that circumstance. Instead of declaring and fighting or getting angry, I'll pause 10 seconds before speaking."

8. Avoid placing blame on others.

When they don't succeed, many people end up finding justifications. Successful people don't hide behind excuses; rather, they view failures as an opportunity to reevaluate and try again. Make it a habit to resist justifications and instead empower yourself to continue pursuing your goal.

9. **Set objectives that benefit others.**

It's crucial to maintain motivation when a goal's path becomes challenging. Those that are successful in accomplishing their goals set

significant accomplishments as their benchmarks. They frequently concentrate on objectives that help others. It's easier to keep moving in the direction of success when you know you're doing well.

10. **Form a healthy habit.**

Although being in shape might seem like a goal in and of itself, it eventually aids in the achievement of your other objectives. Those that are successful appear to have boundless vitality, and they achieve this by maintaining a healthy diet and keeping their bodies active. You give yourself the best chance of success by making wise decisions.

11.Remain modest about your talents.

The people who are most successful in achieving their goals are aware that there is always room for improvement. They may accept assistance and produce achievement repeatedly by being humble and teachable.

Conclusion

Exercise cultivates habits.

When exercise is a regular part of your schedule, it will become a habit. If you're a morning person, schedule your workout before taking a shower. Keep hand weights close by if you typically watch TV in the early evening, so you may perform some repetitions while you catch up on your preferred program.

Ask the professionals: How Do You Form a Habit of Exercise?

So, how exactly do we go about creating a habit, whether it is for exercise or at work? We chose to consult the experts.

Learn their advice on developing wholesome habits and developing the habit of exercising.

Why, in spite of the early psychological benefits, do some people fail to find a purpose for exercise?

For the first time, getting motivated to workout is simple. When we need to find motivation to repeatedly accomplish something, problems typically arise.

It probably won't work every time you try to persuade yourself to workout every day.

Although there are immediate advantages to exercise, such as mood increases, many of these advantages

can only be attained over the long term by engaging in regular activity. This means that maintaining motivation requires choosing exercise over other, sometimes more alluring, options on a regular basis (e.g., watching Netflix). It probably won't always work if you have to persuade yourself to exercise every day (such as when motivation wanes or other things take priority).

Over time, habit might make it simpler to exercise because it simplifies the decision-making process rather than making the activity itself easier. That is, you may "simply do it" out of habit rather than needing to convince yourself to exercise.

Can we form habits in our mind, like

regular exercise?

How to develop the habit of exercising

According to studies, attempting something new twenty days in a row will help you develop a habit (i.e., you do it without thinking or needing to find the motivation).

Automatic (emotional) or reflective motivation is possible (beliefs, intentions).

To create that habit, you must first take into account three important factors. They aid in determining what has to change in order for a habit to be established and are referred to as the COM B Model of Behaviour.

1) **Capability**: Is there something you should start doing right away, such as running?Do you need to start with a different exercise type and work up to it first? Or would you be willing to just dive right in and give it a shot?

2) **Possibility**: Do you, for example, have the proper running shoes?Is this an item you could buy?

3) **Motivation** can be either instinctive (emotional) or intentional (beliefs, intentions).For instance, do you think or feel that this new behavior is good for you?

HOW LONG SHOULD WE CONTINUE SOMETHING NEW TO CREATE A LONG LASTING HABIT?

I won't provide you with the exact

number of times or days you must exercise in order to form a habit. It varies from person to person.

However, habit building often isn't aided by the achievement driven mindset of a countdown of days. Instead, exercisers must discover a method that suits them and fits into their everyday schedules.

www.ingramcontent.com/pod-product-compliance
Lightning Source LLC
Chambersburg PA
CBHW070605160726
48003CB00005B/2125